SPINAL STENOSIS TREATMENT GUIDE

A Definitive step by step guide on the best treatment for Spinal Stenosis

By

Dr. Harvey Donald

Copyright @ 2024.

Table of Contents

PREFACE

This book will literally guide you on what you ought to know about spinal stenosis and its treatment. The book will teach you on the symptoms of spinal stenosis, causes and risk factors of spinal stenosis, tests and diagnosis of spinal stenosis, treatment options for spinal stenosis, surgical options for spinal stenosis, exercises for spinal stenosis, spinal stenosis diet guide and so much more.

CHAPTER ONE

INTRODUCTION

Spinal stenosis is a condition which occurs when the spaces in your spine constrict or narrow as a result of aging, injury, or a medical condition. The process which is generally slow can occur anywhere along the spine. If the narrowing is minimal, no symptoms will occur, although extreme narrowing can compress the spinal canal, causing it to pinch on the spinal cord and nerve roots thus resulting into problems such as *back pain and sciatica.*

Injuries can also result into a narrowed or constricted spinal canal.

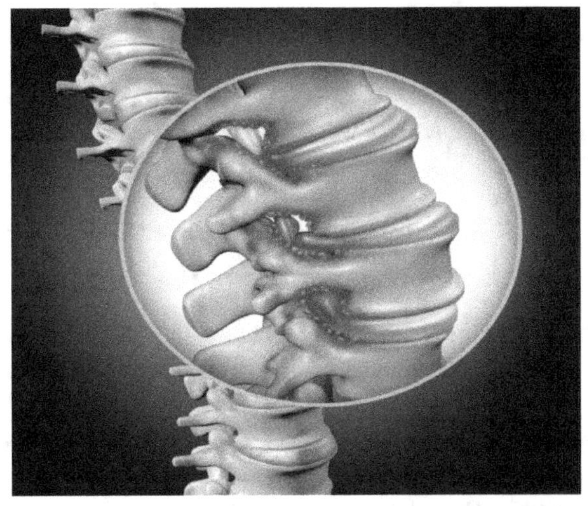

With spinal stenosis, you may develop pain, muscle weakness, tingling, numbness often in the feet and legs as well as other form of symptoms particularly if the spinal cord is compressed.

The vertebrae are 33 bones that connect to form the spinal canal with the spinal canal containing the spinal cord which extends from the base of the skull down through the lower back.

The spinal cord which is a key part of the central nervous system that connects the brain to the body separates out at its base into a bundle of nerve roots. The nerve roots branch out of the spinal canal via gaps in the vertebrae (connected bones).

The spine which offers stability and support to your upper body helps you to twist and turn.

The spinal cord constitutes of spinal nerves, which conduct signals from your brain to the rest of your body with the surrounding bone and tissues constantly protecting the nerves. Damage to the spinal nerves can affect your daily function and activities.

There are various types of spinal stenosis and they include:

(a) **Cervical Spinal Stenosis-** This type of stenosis typically affects the neck.

(b) **Lumbar Spinal Stenosis-** This type of stenosis typically affects the lower back.

(c) **Tandem Spinal Stenosis-** This type of stenosis typically affects at least two (2) areas (parts) of the spine.

(d) **Foraminal Stenosis-** This type of stenosis typically affects the openings in your bones where nerves or vessels normally pass (foramen).

The middle back (thoracic spine) can also develop spinal stenosis, although this is not common.

The most prevalent cause of spinal stenosis is wear-and-tear changes in the spine and individuals who develop this may require surgical options for healing.

Surgery can create more space inside the spine which in turn relieves the symptoms caused by pressure on the spinal cord or nerves. Nevertheless, surgery can not cure arthritis, thus making arthritis pain to continue in the spine.

Spinal stenosis is somewhat common. Degenerative spinal changes affects up to 95% of individuals by the age of 50. Spinal stenosis is one of those changes and for individuals over the age of 65 undergoing spine surgery; lumbar spinal stenosis is the most common form of diagnosis.

CHAPTER TWO

SIGNS AND SYMPTOMS OF SPINAL STENOSIS

Spinal stenosis which normally occurs at the neck and lower back can affect anyone, although it is most common in individuals over the age of 50.

The symptoms of spinal stenosis generally develop over time as nerves become more compressed. Symptoms of spinal stenosis normally depend on which part of the spine is affected.

Nervertheless, if you have spinal stenosis, you might experience symptoms such as:

(a) Numbness and cramps in your legs or buttocks.

(b) Weakness or tingling in the hand, leg, arm, or foot.

(c) Neck pain

(d) Sciatica

(e) Sexual dysfunction

(f) Difficulty in walking

(g) Problems with balance and walking as well as problems with the bowel or bladder

(h) Lower back pain while standing or walking for a long period of time.

In severe and intense cases, an individual may experience partial or complete leg paralysis. This is a medical emergency, and thus the individual should consult the local emergency services instantly.

Sitting in a chair often helps in relieving these symptoms, although the symptoms may return when you stand or walk.

Spinal stenosis can also result into problems with **bladder control, bowel control and sexual function.**

Furthermore, some individuals develop a type of spinal stenosis referred to as *cauda equine syndrome (CES).* The *cauda equine syndrome (CES)* which affects the nerve roots at the base of the spine is a severe condition that can cause permanent paralysis and incontinence if an individual goes without treatment.

Some of the symptoms of cauda equine syndrome (CES) may include:

(a) Weakness in one leg or around both legs
(b) Difficulty in walking and sciatic nerve pain, which travels down one leg.

(c) Loss of sexual function as well as abnormal   bladder/bladder function.

(d) Loss of sensation across the anus, genitals, and inner thighs.

CHAPTER THREE

CAUSES AND RISK FACTORS OF SPINAL STENOSIS

The most prevalent cause of spinal stenosis is aging and individuals over the age of 50 are at a major risk.

Spinal bones are stacked in column from the skull to the tailbone thus protecting the spinal cord, which runs via an opening referred to as the spinal canal.

Some of the health conditions that may contribute to spinal stenosis may include:

(a) **Ankylosing spondylitis-** Ankylosing spondylitis is a form of arthritis that results into chronic inflammation in the spine. Furthermore, it can result into the growth of bone spurs.

(b) **Achondroplasia-** Achondroplasia is a form of dwarfism that interferes with the formation of the bone in the spine as well as other parts of the body.

(c) **Ossification of the posterior longitudinal ligament-** In this health condition, calcium deposits form on the ligament that expends or run through the spinal canal (spinal cavity).

(d) **Congenital spinal stenosis-** This condition happens when you are born with a naturally narrow spinal canal (spinal cavity). Furthermore, this condition is present from birth and it is often the result of having a small spinal canal.

(e) **Scoliosis-** Scoliosis is a sideway curvature or an abnormal lateral curvature of the spine (backbone) that may result from certain genetic conditions, neurological abnormalities, or causes that are unknown.

(f) Osteoarthritis- Osteoarthritis which is a degenerative form of arthritis typically affects the cartilage between vertebrae and cause bone spurs to grow in the spine as an individual ages. Furthermore, the cartilage that shields your joints breaks down. Osteoarthritis is the most prevalent cause of acquired spinal stenosis.

(g) Rheumatoid arthritis- Rheumatoid arthritis is a chronic inflammatory and autoimmune disease that can result into bone damage as well as the development of bone spurs.

(h) Paget's disease of the bone- This is a chronic condition that causes bones to get debilitated and grow bigger than normal.

(i) **Spinal tumors-** These are growths in the tissue that may develop in the spinal canal; induce inflammation as well as cause changes in the surrounding bone. On rare occasions, tumors can form inside the spinal canal.

(j) **Spinal injuries-** Car accidents and other form of trauma can cause spinal bones to break or move out of position resulting to bone fracture. This may cause bone fragments to put pressure on the spinal nerves. Furthermore, swelling of nearby tissue immediately after back surgery can also put pressure on the spinal cord or nerves.

(k) **Thick ligaments-** The strong cord that help connect the bones of your spine together can become stiff and thick over time and again, thick ligaments can push into the spinal canal.

(l) **Herniated disks-** Disks are the soft cushions or shields that act as shock absorbers between your spinal bones and if portion or part of the disk's soft inner material leaks out, it can affect the nerves negatively.

Having excess calcium or fluoride in the body can also result into spinal stenosis.

CHAPTER FOUR

TESTS AND DIAGNOSIS FOR SPINAL STENOSIS

If you have symptoms of spinal stenosis, a physician or a rheumatologist generally begins by taking a medical history, carrying out a physical examination as well as monitoring your movements.

The physician may also order tests to look out for signs of stenosis and other health conditions that may describe your symptoms.

Some of the tests your physician may order include:

(a) *X-ray of the spinal column,* which can help in identifying or detecting osteoarthritic changes. Each X-ray involves a little dose of radiation.

(b) ***Computed tomography, or Magnetic resonance imaging scan*** which can help in detecting or identifying changes to the tissues in and around the spinal canal. The ***Computed tomography scan*** combines X-ray images taken from numerous different angles. The ***Magnetic resonance imaging scan*** makes use of a powerful magnet and radio waves to produce detailed and clear images of hard and soft tissue which in turn help in detecting damage to the disks and ligaments as well as show tumors that may be present.

(c) ***Bone scan*** to check for impairment or growths in the spine

(d) ***Electromyogram*** which makes use of an electrode to evaluate electrical activity in the nerves and muscles.

(e) ***Myelogram test,*** which involves injecting dye into the vertebra column to distinguish between several types of tissues. In a CT myelogram, a contrast dye is injected to outline the spinal cord and nerves which in turn can show herniated disks, tumors and bone spurs.

Furthermore, a physician may also request other kind of tests such as blood tests, to rule different causes of an individual's symptoms.

CHAPTER FIVE

TREATMENT FOR SPINAL STENOSIS

Spinal stenosis treatment generally depends on how severe your symptoms are as well as the symptoms you are experiencing.

Some treatment options may include:

(a) Non-steroidal anti-inflammatory drugs to help in relieving pain.

(b) Physical therapy to help to aid in strengthening and stretching your muscles.

(c) A short procedure of oral corticosteroids to decrease inflammation.

(d) Injections or infusions of cortisone into your spine to help decrease swelling.

(e) Other types of medications if you experience of any form of nerve pain.

Surgery may be recommended if you have severe pain or weakness and other form of treatments that have not worked. Most individuals will be able to address their condition with nonsurgical treatments.

Medications for Spinal stenosis

(a) Antidepressants- Nocturnal doses of tricyclic antidepressants such as *amitriptyline* can help alleviate chronic pain.

(b) Non-steroidal anti-inflammatory drugs- Prescription ***non-steroidal anti-inflammatory drugs*** can help ease pain particularly if common pain relievers don't provide sufficient relief.

(c) Anti-seizure drugs- Some anti-seizure drugs, such as ***gabapentin***

(Gralise, Neurontin) are normally used in mitigating pain caused by impaired or damaged nerves.

(d) Opioids- Medications such as **hydrocodone** *(Hysingla ER)* and **oxycodone** *(Roxicodone, Oxycontin)* can be addictive.

Furthermore, a physical therapist or an exercise therapist can teach you exercises that may help in

- Building up your strength as well as endurance.
- Improving your balance as well as maintaining the flexibility and stability of your spine.

Exercise can be a vital component of spinal stenosis management and the exercise you perform on your own can complement physical therapy.

Try to build an exercise routine around activities that enhances your balance and flexibility or strengthen your core and spine.

Consult a physician or physical therapist first to make sure your at-home exercise routine is safe and adequate. A physical therapist can generally offer a home exercise program to follow during and after physical therapy.

Some of the likely and possible activities may include **short stints of walking, swimming, making use of a stationary bike, modified versions of the moves learnt in physical therapy as well as some yoga moves such as cat-cow or child's pose.**

Steroid shots for Spinal Stenosis

Your nerve roots may become inflamed and swollen at the spots where they are being strained and thus injecting a steroid medication into the space around the strained nerve may help in mitigating the irritation and ease some of the pain.

Nevertheless, steroid shots may not be the ideal choice for spinal stenosis. Some studies have demonstrated that combined injections of steroids and a numbing medicine alleviate back pain no better that just shots of numbing medicine alone.

This is vital since steroids can result into severe side effects. Iterated or repeated steroid injections can debilitate nearby bones, ligaments and tendons. That's why an individual usually must wait many months prior to getting another steroid injection.

Needle technique for thickened ligaments

Occasionally, the ligament at the back of the lumbar spine gets extremely thick. Needle-like tools infused via the skin can discard or remove some of the ligament which in turn can create more space in the spinal canal to decrease pressure on nerve roots. You may be administered medication to help you feel calm during the technique. Nevertheless, numerous individuals can go home same day.

Natural Home remedies for Spinal Stenosis

There are some home remedies as well as complimentary therapies that can help in relieving symptoms of spinal stenosis.

(a) **Cold therapy-** In this procedure, you apply ice or a towel-wrapped cold pact to swollen areas which in turn help in relieving pain and swelling.

(b) **Heat therapy-** This procedure requires the use of a heating pad, warm towel, warm bath, or other heat sources to relax stiff muscles.

(c) Acupuncture

(d) Massage

(e) Yoga

Surgical options for Spinal Stenosis

Individuals with serious pain and weakness that does not respond to other treatments may need surgery. Surgery may also be prescribed by a physician if the condition is literally affecting your ability to walk, control your bowel as well as performing other daily activities.

Various forms or types of surgery are used in treating spinal stenosis and they include:

(a) **Foraminotomy-** Foraminotomy is a form of surgery used in widening the foramen (the parts of the spine where nerve exit/pass through).

(b) **Laminectomy-** This is the most common form of spinal stenosis surgery where the physician or surgeon removes part of the vertebrae (lamina) to provide enough room for the nerves. This surgery eases pressure on the nerves by making enough space around them and in some instances, that bone may need to be connected to close or spinal bones with metal hardware and a bone graft.

(c) **Laminoplasty-** This surgery is performed only on spinal bones in the neck thus making the space within the spinal canal larger by creating a hinge on the lamina. Metal hardware narrows the gap in the opened section or part of the spine.

(d) **Spinal Fusion-** Spinal fusion is generally performed or done in more severe cases, particularly when multiple levels of the spine are involved. The surgeon or physician makes use of bone grafts or metal implants to affix the affected parts of the spine together.

(e) **Spinal decompression-** Spinal decompression which helps to alleviate severe symptoms of spinal stenosis involves removing bony growths and other inflamed tissues from the spinal canal, thus creating enough space for the nerves and spinal cord.

A surgeon or a physician performs spinal decompression as an open spine surgical operation or as a slightly invasive technique, depending on the situation.

The slightly invasive procedure involves a physician inserting a tiny camera and other surgical instruments via a small incision. This technique or method causes less damage to the muscles and soft tissues as it carries a decreased risk of infection.

Nevertheless, in most instances, these surgical operations help decrease symptoms of spinal stenosis, although some individual's symptoms stay the same or get aggravated after surgery.

CHAPTER SIX

EXERCISES FOR SPINAL STENOSIS

If your spinal stenosis results into discomfort; your physician may recommend exercises to decrease or alleviate symptoms. You may be able to build strength, enhance your flexibility via exercise as this may in turn help you to stay active.

Strengthening the core muscles helps in enhancing spinal stenosis symptoms and also, targeting your core strengthens muscles that support your spine, which may relieve your symptoms.

Exercises for spinal stenosis typically focus on changing the position of your spine to help take the pressure off the spinal nerves and this in turn can help in reducing your pain and enhance your general movement.

Exercises for spinal stenosis

(a) Lumbar Flexion exercise in Lying-
To begin your spinal stenosis lumbar flexion exercise movement, carryout the flexion in lying exercise.

Directions

- With your knees bent, lie on your back and gradually bring your knees up to your chest, and grab onto them with your hands.
- Hold onto this position for two seconds and release your knees back to the beginning position.
- Iterate 10 times before proceeding on to another exercise.

(b) Hip and core strengthening exercises- If you develop symptoms of spinal stenosis or have spinal stenosis, *core*

strengthening exercises can help enhance the way the muscles that support your spine work.

The posterior pelvic tilt is an excellent exercise that works your abdominal and hip muscles while stretching your spine and to perform the pelvic tilt:

- Lie on your back with your knees bent and gradually roll your pelvis backward as if you were flattening out your spine.
- Hold onto this position for about 3 seconds and gradually return to the starting position.
- Repeat or iterate 10 times.

*Hip strengthening exercise may help you in enhancing your walking ability. For instance, you could begin with basic **straight leg raises** and then proceed to **advanced hip strengthening***

exercises *with your physical therapist helping you to decide which exercises are best for your particular condition.*

(c) Standing Lumbar Flexion exercises- Standing lumbar flexion is an excellent exercise for people with spinal stenosis.

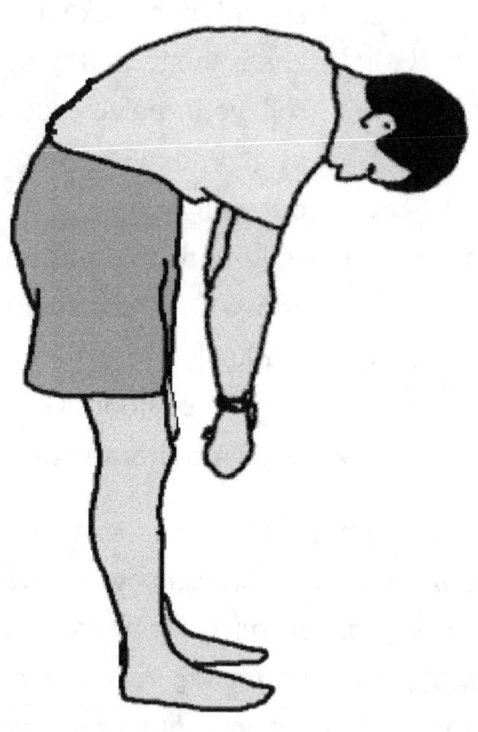

Directions

- Stand with your feet apart and gradually bend yourself forward, reaching towards the floor.
- Hold for about 2 to 3 seconds when you are totally bent and gradually return to the upright standing position.
- Repeat or iterate the exercise for around 10 times.

Seated Lumbar Flexion exercises

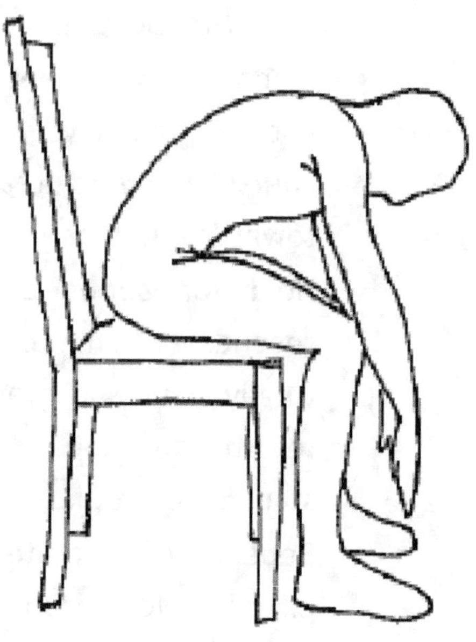

Directions

- With both feet on the floor, sit in a firm chair and gradually bend yourself forward and reach toward the floor.

- Hold the completely bent position for about two seconds and if you need to deepen the stretch, clutch your ankles and give a mild tug.

- After holding the position for two (2) seconds, release and return to the complete, upright seated position and then iterate 10 times and then proceed to the next exercise.

(d) Sustained Lumbar Extension exercise

Directions

- Stand with your feet shoulder-width apart and then support your back and bend backward.
- Hold the position for about 1 minute (60 seconds).

This position may result into an increase in your back pain, as well as leg pain or tingling and if these symptoms subside with 1 minute, this exercise can be added to your lumbar stenosis home regimen.

(e) Plank exercises- Planks are often recommended to individuals who are trying to strengthen their core.

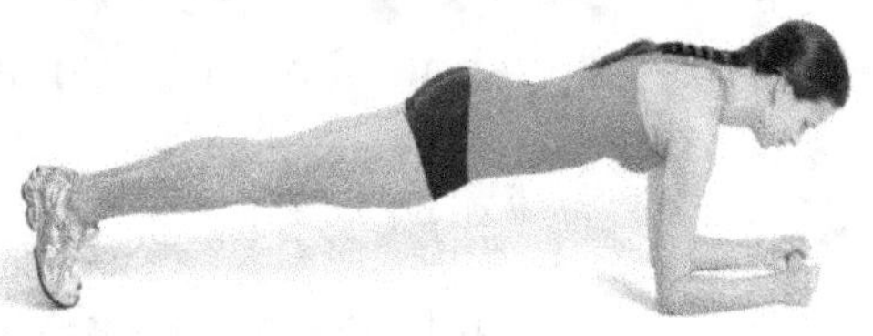

Directions

Traditional plank- With your elbows bent and your hands close to your shoulders, lie on your stomach and lift your body, leaning on your forearms and toes, staying aligned to the floor. Without allowing your hips or stomach sag, hold your body in this position and remain in place for about 30 seconds, and then relax to the floor.

Side plank- With your knees bent and your left elbow directly under your shoulder, lie on your left side and lift your hips, keeping your body straight, balancing on your elbow and knees. Lower your hips and stay in this position for about 10 to 30 seconds. Iterate or repeat this exercise while lying on your right side, leaning on your right elbow.

(f) Knee to chest stretches/exercises

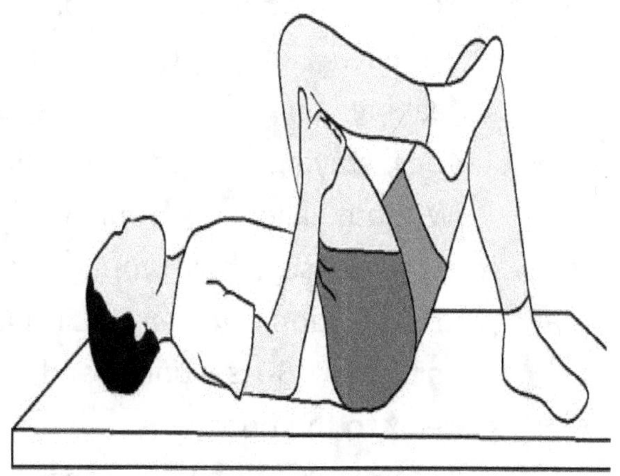

Directions

- Pull both of your knees into your chest and then lie on your back.

- Holding this position for about 30 seconds, clutch your bent knees and then lower your legs.

- Pull only one knee to your chest, keeping the other leg lying flat and then hold your leg behind your knee for 30 seconds and lower the leg.

- Iterate or repeat each of these exercises 5 times and for the single knee stretches, alternate raising each knee to your chest about 5 times.

(g) Standing quadriceps stretches/exercises

Direction

- Stand close to an athletic chair and hold on for support with your right hand.
- Bringing your left foot toward your left butt cheek, bend your left knee.
- With your knee pointing toward the floor, reach your left hand back to clutch your foot.

- Lower your foot, lift your right foot, supporting yourself with your left hand and then iterate or repeat 5 times, alternating left and right.

(h) **Aerobic exercises-** Spinal stenosis is a progressive condition that develops slowly and with debilitating symptoms, you may reduce your level of aerobic activity.

To help manage your spinal stenosis treatment, work with your healthcare professional so that you can begin to integrate aerobic exercise into your routine such as:

- **Walking-** An effective intervention for individuals experiencing lower back pain.

- **Biking-** This helps in positioning your spine in a stenosis-friendly tilted position. It is also an ideal alternative if your symptoms prevent you from walking any form of long distance.

*Note- You should avoid high-impact exercises that involve running and jumping as a result of jolts to the spine and this may include contact sports such as football. Nevertheless, low-impact exercises such as swimming are ideal, although ask your exercise therapist about trying both **extension exercises** (bending back) and **flexion exercises** (bending forward) to build up the spine.*

CHAPTER SEVEN

SPINAL STENOSIS DIET GUIDE

Consuming a healthy diet can also help in relieving numerous symptoms associated with spinal stenosis.

Foods to consume

(a) **Calcium-** Calcium is a mineral that plays a vital role in maintaining strong bones as you tend to grow older. Sources of calcium may include *almonds, dairy products, green leafy vegetables, and wild caught salmon.*

(b) **Healthy proteins-** Healthy proteins play a vital role in healing as well as repairing and maintaining bone and cartilage. Sources of healthy proteins include *fish, eggs, tofu, and lean meats.*

(c) **Vitamin D3-** This is excellent for bone health since it helps you in absorbing calcium. Sources of vitamin D3 may include *cheese, egg yolks, and fatty fish such as tuna, salmon and mackerel. Foods such as orange juice, cereal, soy milk, and some dairy products are also fortified with vitamin D.*

(d) **Magnesium-** Magnesium is a mineral that helps in maintaining bone density and muscle strength. Consume magnesium rich foods such as *avocados, bananas, spinach, brown rice, almonds and broccoli.*

CONCLUSION

Spinal stenosis is a condition which occurs when the spaces in your spine constrict or narrow as a result of aging, injury, or a medical condition. The process which is generally slow can occur anywhere along the spine. If the narrowing is minimal, no symptoms will occur, although extreme narrowing can compress the spinal canal, causing it to pinch on the spinal cord and nerve roots thus resulting into problems such as *back pain and sciatica.*

THE END.

47